CODE FOR OBESITY

HOW TO LOSS WEIGHT IN NO TIME

Unlocking the Path to Sustainable Weight Loss and Wellness

STEVE OPERA

Table of Contents

INTRODUCTION

In today's fast-paced society, obesity has emerged as a grave worldwide health concern that affects millions of people of all ages. Setting realistic objectives, acknowledging the complexity of obesity, and comprehending the significance of efficient weight management are essential first steps to attaining quick and long-lasting weight reduction. In an effort to solve the obesity puzzle and open the door to a healthier, happier, and more satisfying existence, this essay examines these three key factors.

UNDERSTANDING OBESITY

An excessive buildup of bodily fat characterizes the complex disorder known as obesity. Although obesity is frequently linked to aesthetic issues, it is important to realize that it affects much more than just looks. The intricate interaction of genetic, environmental, behavioral, and metabolic variables causes this illness. Its growth may be influenced by poor food choices, sedentary lifestyles, and genetic predispositions. Additionally, obesity is frequently linked to an increased risk of a number of health issues, including as diabetes, heart disease, and several types of cancer.

A crucial first step in the process of losing weight is realizing the root reasons of obesity. It helps people to make wise choices and personalize their weight loss plans to deal with the underlying issues that are unique to their situation.

THE IMPORTANCE OF WEIGHT MANAGEMENT

Effective weight control involves more than just losing extra weight for aesthetic benefits. It aims to promote general health and wellbeing. When we start down the path of weight management, our goals are to increase physical fitness, lower the risk of obesity-related health problems, and improve overall quality of life.

In addition to raising self-esteem, a healthy weight also eases the strain on our joints, increases energy, and supports mental wellness. The ability to regulate one's weight gives people the strength to take charge of their life and implement lasting, beneficial changes to their daily routines.

SETTING REALISTIC GOALS

It might be alluring to want to lose weight rapidly, but it's important to approach the process with a realistic outlook. Although intense workout routines and crash diets may produce short-term gains, they are frequently unsustainable and hazardous over the long term. A good weight management approach must include realistic weight loss targets.

Realistic objectives should take into account a person's age, metabolism, and personal responsibilities. They should be attainable and long-lasting, emphasizing forward movement rather than sudden, abrupt shifts. People may stay motivated, monitor their progress, and celebrate their victories along the way by setting achievable goals.

In conclusion, a thorough understanding of obesity, awareness of the significance of weight management, and the development of attainable objectives are the first steps in solving the mystery of obesity and attaining quick weight reduction. People may start a lasting and successful weight reduction journey by addressing these core issues, which will ultimately improve their general health and quality of life. The subtitle is "Cracking the Code for Obesity: Achieving Rapid Weight Loss"

CHAPTER ONE

NUTRITION AND DIET
THE ROLE OF NUTRITION IN WEIGHT LOSS

Any successful weight loss plan must start with good nutrition. Beyond calorie tracking and extreme diets, it goes deeper. A caloric deficit is created to encourage weight reduction while maintaining the proper balance of nutrients for the body's general health. This equilibrium guarantees that crucial vitamins, minerals, and other nutrients are provided even if calorie consumption is decreased.

CREATING A BALANCED DIET PLAN

Healthy and quick weight reduction is built on a balanced food plan. It consists of a range of meals from several dietary categories to make sure the body gets all the necessary nutrients. Fruits, vegetables, lean meats, whole grains, and healthy fats are important elements of a nutrition plan that is balanced. Portion management is also essential since it helps sustain a calorie deficit by preventing overeating.

COUNTING CALORIES: A GUIDE

Calorie counting is a popular weight-management strategy. People can better regulate their food intake by measuring their calorie intake and determining their daily caloric needs. Instead of turning to excessive calorie restriction, which may be ineffective, it is crucial to establish a sustained caloric deficit. Both the number and the type of calories consumed—such as those from nutrient-dense foods—are crucial.

THE IMPACT OF MACRONUTRIENTS

Carbohydrates, proteins, and fats, or macronutrients, are key in the process of losing weight. Each performs a certain job in the body. Proteins help with muscle upkeep and repair, while lipids are necessary for general health. Carbohydrates offer energy. The proper distribution of these macronutrients is ensured by a well-balanced diet, with a focus on whole grains for carbs, lean sources for proteins, and healthy fats from foods like nuts and avocados.

SMART FOOD CHOICES

A successful weight reduction journey depends on making wise eating decisions. It's important to choose nutrient-dense meals over processed or sugary alternatives. Any diet plan should include whole grains, lean meats, and lots of fruits and vegetables. To lose weight quickly, it's also important to restrict the intake of high-calorie, low-nutrient foods and stay away from sugary beverages. In conclusion, quick weight loss with food and nutrition necessitates a thorough strategy. To do this, you must comprehend how nutrition affects weight reduction, design a balanced meal plan, calculate calories sustainably, take into account the effects of macronutrients, and constantly make healthy food choices. People can discover the secret to effective and long-lasting weight loss by paying attention to these factors and tailoring dietary solutions to individual needs. "Cracking the Code for Obesity: Achieving Rapid Weight Loss through Nutrition and Diet," book title.

CHAPTER TWO

EXERCISE AND PHYSICAL ACTIVITY

Exercise and physical activity are effective methods for obtaining quick weight loss. In the context of weight control, this section will examine five important components of exercise.

BENEFITS OF EXERCISE FOR WEIGHT LOSS

There are several advantages to exercise while trying to lose weight. First of all, it raises the overall daily energy expenditure, assisting in establishing the calorie deficit required for weight loss. Additionally, regular exercise increases metabolism, which makes it simpler to sustain weight reduction. Additionally, it has a beneficial effect on mental health, lowering stress and improving general wellbeing, which may help with weight control indirectly.

FINDING AN EXERCISE ROUTINE THAT WORKS

Finding a routine that is pleasurable and sustainable is one of the biggest obstacles to keeping up with a workout program. It's crucial to select activities that fit with individual tastes and lifestyles. The secret is to pick a fitness regimen that you enjoy and can commit to on a regular basis, whether it's running, cycling, dancing, or team sports.

CARDIOVASCULAR WORKOUTS

Exercises that increase heart health and burn calories are beneficial. When coupled with a healthy diet, exercises like jogging, swimming, and cycling increase heart rate and aid in fat reduction. Maintaining a regular cardiovascular exercise plan is crucial to maximizing the effects of weight reduction, gradually increasing intensity and duration over time.

STRENGTH TRAINING FOR FAT LOSS

Resistance training, often known as strength training, is essential for weight loss. These exercises aid in the development of lean muscle, which raises metabolism and causes the body to burn more calories even when at rest. Furthermore, muscle is more compact than fat, giving the illusion of being slimmer. Both aerobic and strength training should be a part of a well-rounded workout regimen.

STAYING ACTIVE THROUGHOUT THE DAY

Physical activity encompasses many aspects of daily life and is not only reserved for regimented workouts. Including extra activity in your regular routines will help you lose weight in a big way. Taking the stairs, traveling by foot or bicycle to work, and getting up or stretching after extended periods of sitting can all assist to raise daily energy expenditure.

In order to lose weight quickly, exercise and physical activity are essential steps to do. In order to defeat obesity and achieve lasting, beneficial changes in weight management, it is essential to understand the many advantages of exercise, find a routine that you enjoy and can stick with, incorporate cardiovascular and strength training, and stay active throughout the day.

CHAPTER THREE

LIFESTYLE CHANGES

For sustained success and speedy weight loss, lifestyle is a key factor. Let's look at five essential lifestyle elements that might support people in their quest for improved weight management:

THE POWER OF SLEEP

Weight reduction requires a good night's sleep. The body heals itself when sleeping deeply and regulates hunger and appetite hormones. Lack of sleep can interfere with these functions, increasing the desire for unhealthy meals and decreasing the desire to exercise. Effective weight control depends on putting a high priority on excellent sleep hygiene, which includes aiming for 7-9 hours of high-quality sleep each night.

STRESS AND WEIGHT MANAGEMENT

Losing weight can be significantly hampered by stress. Cortisol, a hormone that is released by the body in response to stress, can cause fat to be stored, particularly in the abdominal region. Learning stress-reduction strategies like mindfulness, yoga, or meditation can improve good weight control by lowering stress levels.

BUILDING HEALTHY HABITS

The most positive adjustments to a lifestyle occur when they become ingrained. Sustainable weight reduction may be achieved by developing healthy habits including regular exercise, meal planning, and mindful eating. It is crucial to concentrate on tiny, doable adjustments that may be incorporated into everyday life since habits are created by repeated action over time.

MINDFUL EATING AND PORTION CONTROL

During meals, one should be totally present, enjoy each bite, and pay attention to their body's hunger and fullness signs. This strategy can discourage binge eating and encourage a better connection with food. Another crucial component of mindful eating is portion management since it limits calorie intake. Measure your meals and use smaller dishes as efficient portion management techniques.

COPING WITH CRAVINGS

A frequent obstacle to weight loss is cravings for unhealthy meals. It's crucial to know the difference between actual hunger and cravings brought on by emotions or stress.

Having wholesome alternatives on hand and using moderation might aid people in making better decisions when cravings arise. Recognizing that occasional indulgences are appropriate and a necessary component of a balanced weight-management strategy is also crucial.

In summary, altering one's lifestyle is essential for defeating obesity and attaining quick weight reduction. A thorough approach to weight management should include understanding the importance of sleep, managing stress, forming healthy habits, practicing mindful eating and portion control, and learning how to deal with cravings. Individuals can increase their chances of attaining effective and long-lasting weight loss by addressing certain lifestyle variably.

CHAPTER FOUR

WEIGHT LOSS STRATEGIES

There are many different weight loss methods available, and people frequently have a wide range of choices. It's critical to discern between practical, long-term solutions and fad diets or supplements, which may promise immediate outcomes but frequently fall short. Here are the top five methods for losing weight to think about.

FAD DIETS VS. SUSTAINABLE WEIGHT LOSS

Fad diets frequently guarantee quick weight reduction but are usually hazardous in the long run. They frequently emphasize extreme caloric restriction or the banning of whole food categories. On the other hand, maintaining weight reduction that is balanced and long-lasting requires making modifications to one's food and lifestyle. Fad diets are less successful and even dangerous since they can result in nutritional deficits, muscle loss, and rebound weight gain.

INTERMITTENT FASTING: A CLOSER LOOK

An eating habit known as intermittent fasting cycles between periods of eating and fasting. As a result of its potential advantages for weight reduction and general health, this tactic has grown in favor. While intermittent fasting can be successful for some, it might not be the best option for everyone. The secret is to pick a strategy that suits each person's tastes and demands and is long-lasting.

KETO DIET AND ITS EFFECTIVENESS

A low-carb, high-fat diet called the ketogenic (keto) diet has been advocated for quick weight reduction. By triggering a condition of ketosis, when the body burns fat for energy, it may be beneficial in the short term. However, not everyone should follow the ketogenic diet, and more research is needed to determine its long-term consequences. It can cause nutritional shortages and is sometimes challenging to sustain over long.

THE ROLE OF SUPPLEMENTS

Dietary supplements, such as protein powders, vitamins, and minerals, can help with weight reduction, especially if there are nutrient deficits. They do not, however, work as a magic bullet for weight loss on their own. It's doubtful that using supplements only would result in long-term weight loss without also changing your food and lifestyle.

THE TRUTH ABOUT WEIGHT LOSS PILLS

Weight-management aids like tablets or pharmaceuticals are made for that purpose, but they should only be taken with a doctor's prescription. In situations of obesity or when dietary adjustments have failed, they are frequently given. Scientific proof of the effectiveness of over-the-counter weight reduction drugs is sometimes lacking, and they can be dangerous.

In conclusion, there are many various routes to losing weight, and it's important to distinguish between safe methods and possibly dangerous fad diets, supplements, or medications. Making healthy, long-term adjustments to food and lifestyle that can be sustained over time is often required for successful weight loss. It is frequently a good decision to get advice from a licensed dietician or healthcare expert to guarantee a secure and successful weight reduction journey.

CHAPTER FIVE

TRACKING PROGRESS

A crucial part of any weight reduction plan is tracking progress. It inspires people, aids in maintaining focus, and enables modifications as needed. Four essential components for monitoring weight control progress are listed below:

THE IMPORTANCE OF MONITORING YOUR WEIGHT

A crucial tool for evaluating your weight reduction journey's success is routinely keeping track of your weight. It enables you to comprehend how your dietary and lifestyle adjustments have affected you. But it's important to remember that your total health encompasses more than simply your weight. Fluctuations are common, and the scale's numbers might fluctuate due to things like water retention, muscle growth, and hormone changes. It's more crucial to take long-term patterns into account than daily variations.

SETTING MILESTONES AND CELEBRATING SUCCESS

Setting milestones, or more manageable objectives, is a good method to monitor development and keep motivation high. Make the overall result more achievable by dividing it into smaller, more manageable steps. Celebrating your victories along the road may increase motivation and strengthen constructive habits. These milestones may include attaining physical objectives, decreasing a specific amount of weight, or following a healthy eating regimen for a predetermined period of time.

APPS AND TOOLS FOR WEIGHT TRACKING

There are several applications and tools available to assist people keep track of their progress. These tools let you keep track of your weight over time, track your activity, and log your meals. Numerous other characteristics, like goal-setting, tracking your diet, and even social support networks, make them useful tools for healthy weight management.

THE ROLE OF A SUPPORT SYSTEM

Having a support system may be quite helpful while trying to lose weight. Family, close friends, or support groups can all offer help. You may maintain accountability and motivation by telling people about your success and obstacles. Additionally, talking to someone about your objectives and disappointments can offer emotional support and motivation.

In conclusion, measuring progress is an essential part of losing weight quickly and keeping up a healthy lifestyle. You may increase your chances of success by regularly checking your weight, establishing goals and celebrating your achievements, using apps and tools for tracking your weight, and leaning on a support network. Individuals can improve their odds of achieving their weight reduction objectives and maintaining long-term good improvements by putting these ideas into practice.

CHAPTER SIX

STAYING MOTIVATED

Maintaining motivation when trying to lose weight is crucial for getting quick and long-lasting results. The following four essential elements can help you stay motivated:

STAYING COMMITTED TO YOUR WEIGHT LOSS JOURNEY

The key to a successful weight reduction journey is commitment. It's crucial to frequently remind yourself of the motivations behind why you initially embarked on the path in order to stay dedicated. Consider your health objectives, the advantages of losing weight, or the beneficial effects it will have on your life while you do this. Making a vision board or a list of goals might be useful as a written or visual reminder of your commitment to stay on track.

OVERCOMING PLATEAUS

The typical occurrence of weight reduction plateaus might be discouraging. It's crucial to keep in mind that reaching a plateau is a normal part of the trip when you do. Instead of getting frustrated, take the opportunity presented by plateaus to reconsider your strategy. You might have to change your eating habits, exercise regimen, or other components of your weight reduction plan. Remember that breaking through plateaus is a sign of development, and be patient and persistent.

LEARNING FROM SETBACKS

Any attempt to lose weight will inevitably include setbacks and mistakes. Consider them chances to learn and grow as opposed to failures. Determine measures to avoid the setback from occurring again by analyzing the events that led to it. It's important to regard failures as transient roadblocks on the way to your objectives rather than being overly harsh on yourself.

STAYING INSPIRED

Inspiration may originate from a variety of places. Look for role models who have attained their weight loss objectives effectively and take advice from them. Join weight loss support groups, follow motivational fitness and health accounts on social media, and read success stories. You can stay motivated and inspired by surrounding yourself with inspiring people.

In conclusion, maintaining motivation throughout your weight reduction journey is crucial for obtaining quick and long-lasting outcomes. You may retain the motivation required to achieve your weight reduction objectives by being dedicated, overcoming plateaus, learning from setbacks, and seeking inspiration from a variety of sources. Keep in mind that while the trip may have its ups and downs, you can stay focused and eventually achieve with the correct attitude and support.

CHAPTER SEVEN

HEALTHY EATING RECIPE
is essential to preserving health and avoiding a number of chronic illnesses. The following explains the important components you mentioned.

IMPORTANCE OF A BALANCED DIET:
A balanced diet consists of a range of foods from each food category in the appropriate amounts. It guarantees that you obtain the vitamins, minerals, and nutrients your body need for optimum operation. This is why eating a balanced diet is so important:

- **NUTRIENT INTAKE:** You may get a variety of nutrients, such as carbs, proteins, fats, vitamins, and minerals, by eating a balanced diet. Every vitamin has a distinct purpose in the operations of your body.

- **ENERGY LEVELS:** Eating a balanced diet gives you the energy you need for everyday tasks. Energy imbalances can result from consuming too many calories from one food type and not enough from another.

- **WEIGHT MANAGEMENT:** Weight management may benefit from it. You can gain weight if you consume more calories than your body requires, but you can lose weight if you consume less calories.

- **DISEASE PREVENTION:** A healthy diet lowers the chance of developing long-term conditions including diabetes, heart disease, and some types of cancer.

TIPS FOR MEAL PLANNING AND PORTION CONTROL:

To have a balanced diet and limit calorie consumption, meal planning and portion management are crucial. Here are a few pointers:

• Arrange Your Meals: Arrange your snacks and meals in advance. This can assist you in avoiding rash, unwise decisions and helping you make healthier decisions.

• Use Smaller dishes: Eating less and controlling portion sizes are two benefits of using smaller dishes.

• Examine Labels: To learn about nutritional content and portion proportions, read food labels carefully.

Eat mindfully by taking your time, enjoying every mouthful, and paying attention to your body's signals of hunger and fullness.

• Divide Your Plate: To guarantee a healthy dinner, divide your plate into pieces for various dietary groups, such as veggies, lean meats, and whole grains.

ADVICE ON MAKING HEALTHIER FOOD CHOICES:

Choosing foods that are high in good fats, added sugars, and empty calories, while avoiding those that are high in bad fats, is the key to making better meal choices. Here are some pointers:

• Go with Whole Foods: Choose entire foods with little to no processing, such as nuts, fruits, vegetables, whole grains, and lean meats.

LIMIT SUGARY AND PROCESSED FOODS: Limit your use of highly processed meals, sugary drinks, and sugary snacks since they frequently lack important nutrients.

OPT FOR LEAN PROTEINS: Limit red and processed meats and choose for lean protein sources such beans, tofu, fish, and chicken.

HEALTHY FATS: Minimize saturated and trans fats and increase sources of heart-healthy fats, such as nuts, avocados, and olive oil.

HYDRATION: Limit sugary beverages and sip lots of water.

- Moderation: In moderation, indulge in sweets and less nutritious meals.

Keep in mind that each person may have different dietary demands depending on their age, degree of exercise, and health. A licensed dietician or other healthcare expert can help you build a customized plan that fits your objectives and needs.

CONCLUSION

YOUR PERSONALIZED CODE FOR OBESITY

A tailored strategy is needed to combat obesity and lose weight quickly. For obesity, you have a unique personal code. It means understanding the underlying reasons behind your weight gain and figuring out which approaches work best for your body type and lifestyle. Being conscious of yourself and making a commitment to creating a customized plan that addresses the root causes of your obesity is the first step in this process. By acknowledging your own challenges and strengths, you may make your weight loss journey as fruitful and durable as possible.

ACHIEVING SUSTAINABLE WEIGHT LOSS

While rapid weight loss is a commendable goal, sustainability should also be considered. Long-term success lies not just in quickly dropping excess weight but in consistently sustaining a better weight and lifestyle over time.

Sustainable weight loss is all about making long-term changes to your diet, level of physical activity, and overall well-being. It means finding a way to live a full life while prioritizing your health. Sustainability is an ongoing process that requires persistence, as well as adaptability to changing circumstances.

A HEALTHY FUTURE

Ultimately, figuring out the obesity conundrum will result in a happier and healthier future. This journey starts with rapid weight loss. By addressing the numerous aspects of obesity, including nutrition, exercise, lifestyle modifications, and the crucial role of motivation and support, you may enhance your health, elevate your self-esteem, and build a better future. Maintaining a healthy weight and lifestyle reduces your risk of obesity-related health issues, enhances your overall wellness, and opens the door to a life full of energy and joy.

In summary, breaking the obesity code entails adopting a thorough and customized approach to rapid weight loss while prioritizing long-term health and pleasure. Making long-lasting changes, keeping an eye on the future, and acknowledging your own talents and weaknesses might lead to a better, more fulfilling existence.